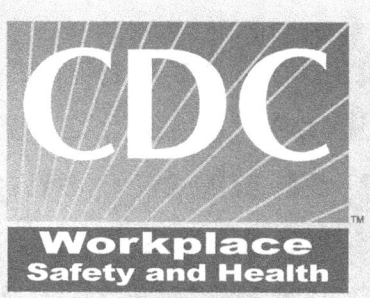

Determining Base Camp Personnel Exposures to Carbon Monoxide during Wildland Fire Suppression Activities – California

Robert E. McCleery, MSPH, CIH
Anthony Almazan, MD
Chad H. Dowell, MS, CIH
John Snawder, PhD, DABT

Health Hazard Evaluation Report
HETA 2008-0245-3127
May 2011

DEPARTMENT OF HEALTH AND HUMAN SERVICES
Centers for Disease Control and Prevention

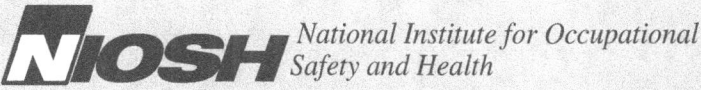

National Institute for Occupational Safety and Health

The employer shall post a copy of this report for a period of 30 calendar days at or near the workplace(s) of affected employees. The employer shall take steps to insure that the posted determinations are not altered, defaced, or covered by other material during such period. [37 FR 23640, November 7, 1972, as amended at 45 FR 2653, January 14, 1980].

CONTENTS

ABBREVIATIONS

ACGIH®	American Conference of Governmental Industrial Hygienists
A/C	Air-conditioning
BEI®	Biological exposure index
CFR	Code of Federal Regulations
CMD	Command
CO	Carbon monoxide
COHb	Carboxyhemoglobin
COMM	Communications
EPA	Environmental Protection Agency
GA	General area
HHE	Health hazard evaluation
IDLH	Immediately dangerous to life and health
NAAQS	National Ambient Air Quality Standard
NAICS	North American Industry Classification System
NIOSH	National Institute for Occupational Safety and Health
OEL	Occupational exposure limit
OSHA	Occupational Safety and Health Administration
PBZ	Personal breathing zone
PEL	Permissible exposure limit
ppm	Parts per million
REL	Recommended exposure limit
STEL	Short-term exposure limit
TLV®	Threshold limit value
TWA	Time-weighted average
WEEL	Workplace environmental exposure limits
WHO	World Health Organization

HIGHLIGHTS OF THE NIOSH HEALTH HAZARD EVALUATION

The National Institute for Occupational Safety and Health (NIOSH) received a request for a health hazard evaluation (HHE) at a base camp supporting the Siskiyou and Ukonom fires in the Klamath National Forest, California. Federal agency managers submitted the request due to concerns about carbon monoxide (CO) exposures of personnel working at base camps who support firefighters during wildland fire suppression activities.

What NIOSH Did

- We evaluated the base camp in August 2008.
- We measured base camp employee's exposure to CO in the air and blood. CO in the blood was measured as carboxyhemoglobin (COHb).
- We measured temperature, relative humidity, and dew point temperatures in the base camp.

What NIOSH Found

- Most base camp employees' CO exposure levels were very low.
- Some base camp employees' CO exposure levels were over peak occupational exposure limits.
- Most COHb measurements were very low. Three out of 19 base camp employees who did not smoke had COHb measurements that were slightly elevated.

What Managers Can Do

- Develop a program to measure base camp employees' exposure to CO and particulates.
- Think about developing CO and particulate action levels for use in future fire events. If used, make sure to account for extended work shifts.
- Implement a program to raise awareness about heat stress.
- Limit the number of employees working extended work shifts. If extended work shifts are needed, make sure these employees get adequate rest and recovery time.

What Employees Can Do

- Avoid working near sources of CO. Other sources of CO in the base camp include gasoline- and diesel-powered vehicles and equipment and cigarette smoke.
- Tell your supervisor if you feel weak, nauseated, excessively fatigued, confused, or irritable. These are signs of heat illness.
- Drink plenty of fluids to prevent heat-related illness

Overall, CO air concentrations and employee COHb measurements were low. However, some peak CO concentrations exceeded relevant OELs. Although not directly comparable to the ACGIH BEI because of the use of 16-hour work shifts, some nonsmoking employees met or exceeded a COHb measurement of 3.5%. We recommend developing a base camp air monitoring program for particulates and CO, establishing a heat stress awareness program, and limiting extended work shifts.

In July 2008, NIOSH received a request for an HHE at a base camp supporting the Siskiyou and Ukonom fires in the Klamath National Forest, California. Federal agency managers submitted the request due to concerns about CO exposure among personnel who work in the base camp supporting wildland firefighters during fire suppression activities. Headaches were listed as the primary health concern.

On August 13–14, 2008, NIOSH investigators conducted PBZ air monitoring for CO exposure and measured blood COHb levels for 19 nonsmoking forestry personnel and contractors and performed GA air sampling for CO in the base camp. Employees' average work shift CO exposures were low (< 6 ppm). However, peak CO concentrations exceeded OELs; 7 of 19 (37%) exceeded the ACGIH excursion limit of 125 ppm, 5 of 19 (26%) exceeded the NIOSH ceiling limit of 200 ppm, and 4 of 19 (21%) exceeded the 1000 ppm upper limit of the instrument (approaching the 1200 ppm NIOSH IDLH level for < 1 minute). The GA monitors located throughout the base camp indicated average CO concentrations of less than 2 ppm with a peak reading of 20 ppm.

Over the 2-day period, 19 nonsmoking employees had COHb measurements taken. Although not directly comparable to the ACGIH BEI (end of shift, 8-hour COHb measurement of 3.5%), 3 of the 19 (16%) nonsmoking employees met or exceeded a COHb measurement of 3.5%, an indicator of a 25 ppm, 8-hour TWA CO exposure. Only one of these employees had a corresponding peak PBZ air CO concentration exceeding the ACGIH excursion limit and none had a corresponding peak PBZ air CO concentration that exceeded the NIOSH ceiling limit. The levels of COHb we found among employees at the base camp have not been documented to cause symptoms that can result from short-term, higher levels of CO exposure. However, the combination of consecutive 16-hour work shifts, continuous exposure to forest fire smoke, and hot environmental conditions could explain headaches reported in the HHE request.

Summary
(CONTINUED)

NIOSH investigators recommend developing a base camp air monitoring program for particulates and CO and limiting the number of personnel working extended shifts as well as the frequency and duration of extended work shifts. We also recommend developing CO and particulate action levels for use during future fire events, taking into consideration employee extended work shifts. A program should also be established to increase base camp personnel's awareness of heat stress.

Keywords: NAICS 924120 (Administration of Conservation Programs), carbon monoxide, CO, carboxyhemoglobin, COHb, base camp, firefighter, wildland forest fire

INTRODUCTION

In July 2008, NIOSH received a request for an HHE at a base camp supporting the Siskiyou and Ukonom fires in the Klamath National Forest, California, during the summer of 2008. Federal agency managers submitted the HHE request because of their concern about potential CO exposures among the personnel working in base camps supporting wildland firefighters during fire suppression activities.

In response to this request, NIOSH investigators conducted an investigation at the base camp on August 13 and 14, 2008. The investigation included GA and PBZ CO air monitoring of forestry personnel and contractors and monitoring of COHb, a biological indicator of CO exposure. This report summarizes our evaluation and provides recommendations for a more healthy work environment for base camp personnel.

Background

Klamath National Forest covers approximately 1.7 million acres in northern California and southern Oregon [USFS 2008]. The forest consists of Ponderosa pine, Douglas fir, sub-alpine fir, and mixed conifer. The Siskiyou and Ukonom forest fires began by lightning strikes in late June 2008. Combining all fires in the area, approximately 200,000 acres burned.

The base camp was located in California in the Klamath River Valley of the Klamath National Forest. This base camp housed the incident command post and was a firefighter staging area for fire suppression operations. The base camp included parking, daily briefing, and crew camping areas (personal tents and sleeping trailers); facilities for dining and showering; laundry and medical services; supply dispersal; vehicle inspection, fueling, and washing areas; and tents and trailers for administrative services, such as communications, planning, logistics, safety, and finance. Diesel generators provided power for tents, trailers, air-conditioning (window A/C units, swamp coolers, and trailer-mounted A/C units), and other base camp equipment.

At the base camp, forestry and contractor personnel and firefighters were grouped into incident management teams consisting of command, supply, medical, communications, and support services. Support services included caterers, camp crew, ground, latrine, shower, and camp security. Base camp personnel worked up to 16-hour shifts. The base camp closed on September 26, 2008.

ASSESSMENT

We measured CO air concentrations on 19 nonsmoking employees (communication, command, medical, resource, and supply staff; caterers; reefers; and mechanics) during the entire 16-hour work shift on August 13, 2008; during the overnight period to evaluate CO concentrations while they slept in their tents (monitors remained beside them); and 6–8 hours during the work shift on August 14, 2008. Additionally, we placed 13 GA CO monitors in base camp locations such as the security area (south), tent camp areas, and various administration tents/trailers.

In association with measuring CO air concentrations, we collected noninvasive measurements of COHb on nonsmokers using a pulse CO-oximeter. We collected these measurements close to the beginning of each work shift, at various times during the work shift, and at the end of the work shift. We excluded current smokers from this measurement since smokers have been shown to have elevated background COHb levels.

We used a weather station to collect climate information (temperature, relative humidity, dew point, and other variables) at the base camp during the entire evaluation.

You can find additional details about these sampling methods in Appendix A and a discussion of OELs and adverse health effects from CO exposure in Appendix B.

Carbon Monoxide in Air

Table 1 provides a summary of real-time PBZ CO air sampling results, while Appendix C, Table C1, presents each individual's PBZ CO air sampling results for the August 13, 2008, work shift, the overnight period, and 6–8 hours of the August 14, 2008, work shift. As Table 1 indicates, the employees' average CO exposures over their work shift were low (< 6 ppm), but some peak CO concentrations were above relevant OELs. Seven of 19 (37%) peak CO exposures exceeded the ACGIH excursion limit of 125 ppm, 5 of 19 (26%) exceeded the NIOSH ceiling limit of 200 ppm, and 4 of 19 (21%) exceeded the 1000 ppm upper limit of the instrument (approaching the 1200 ppm NIOSH IDLH level for < 1 minute). The overnight CO air sampling results provided in Table C1 also indicate low average concentrations of CO (range: 0.12–5.7 ppm). Appendix D, Figures D1–D7 graphically present the real-time CO concentration data for each individual with peak exposures above relevant OELs.

Table 1. Base camp personnel – summary of CO concentrations (ppm) from August 13–14, 2008.

Job	N (shifts)	1st Shift*		Overnight*†		2nd Shift*	
		Avg.	Peak	Avg.	Peak	Avg.	Peak
Caterer	3 (6)	2.6	107	2.5	> 1000‡§	2.1	28
Command	2 (4)	1.1	12	1.1	2.9	2.0	74
Communications¶	2 (3)	2.8	> 1000‡§	1.5	15	2.4	8.6
Mechanic¶	2 (4)	4.8	> 1000‡§**	2.2	7.3	3.2	72
Medical	1 (2)	2.7	49	1.3	3.9	1.5	8.0
Reefer¶	3 (3)	2.6	> 1000‡§	0.30	22	—	—
Resource	1 (2)	2.3	141‡	0.57	5.8	1.9	15
Supply/Logistics	1 (2)	1.1	8.6	1.4	5.5	2.0	15
Supply	3 (6)	1.1	45	2.0	80	3.0	128‡
Weed Wash	1 (1)	—	—	—	—	5.4	40

N = Number of employees (number of total work shifts)

* = Approximate duration – 1st shift (16 hours), overnight (8 hours), 2nd shift (monitored 6–8 hours)

† = Employees kept their CO monitor beside them in their tent while they slept.

‡ = Exceeded the ACGIH excursion limit of 125 ppm

§ = Exceeded the NIOSH ceiling limit of 200 ppm

¶ = 1 of 2 communications employees had 2nd shift data; 1 of 2 mechanics and 2 of 3 reefers had overnight data.

** = Both mechanics exceeded ACGIH excursion and NIOSH ceiling limits (423 ppm and > 1000 ppm).

RESULTS
(CONTINUED)

Table C2 provides the real-time CO concentrations of the GA monitors placed in numerous areas in and around the base camp. These GA monitors indicated average CO concentrations of less than 3 ppm, with the highest peak reading of 20 ppm in the east end of the base camp. Although EPA does not have a 24-hour limit for CO, the average CO concentrations of these GA monitors are well under the EPA NAAQS 8-hour limit of 9 ppm. Figure 1 provides real-time CO concentration data from the north end of the base camp over the entire evaluation period. The CO concentrations measured in this area are similar to the other GA locations and indicate that the visual buildup of smoke in the base camp (Figures 2–4) does not equate to a high CO concentration in the monitored areas.

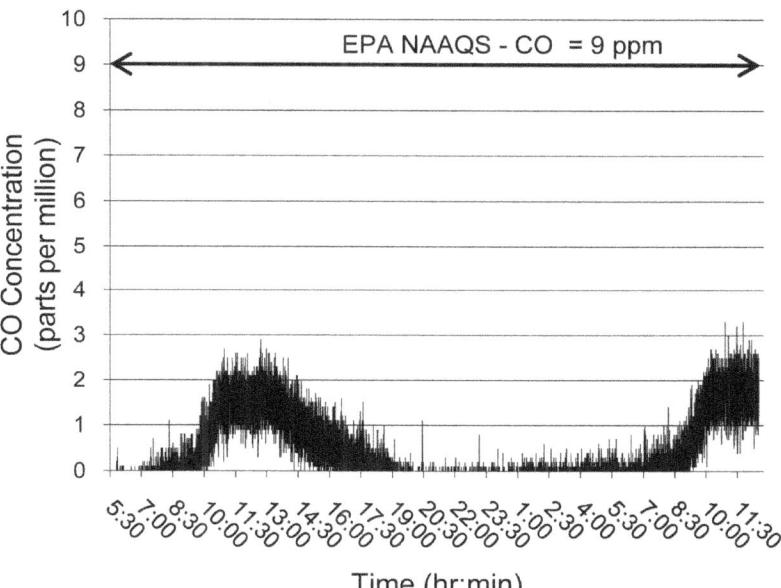

Figure 1. Outdoor CO concentrations at the base camp's north end on August 13–14, 2008.

Figures 2–4 illustrate the smoke buildup in the base camp during our evaluation. Figures 2 and 3 are photographs taken in the same location and looking in the same direction only a few hours apart (approximately 8:30 a.m. and 10:00 a.m.). Smoke buildup in the valley where the base camp was located is clearly visible in these figures. The far mountain range is visible in Figure 2, but not as easily discernable in Figure 3. Additionally, the smoke had settled deeper into the valley by midmorning as seen in Figure 3. Figure 4 is the base camp in the early morning hours (approximately 7:30 a.m.) on August 14, 2008.

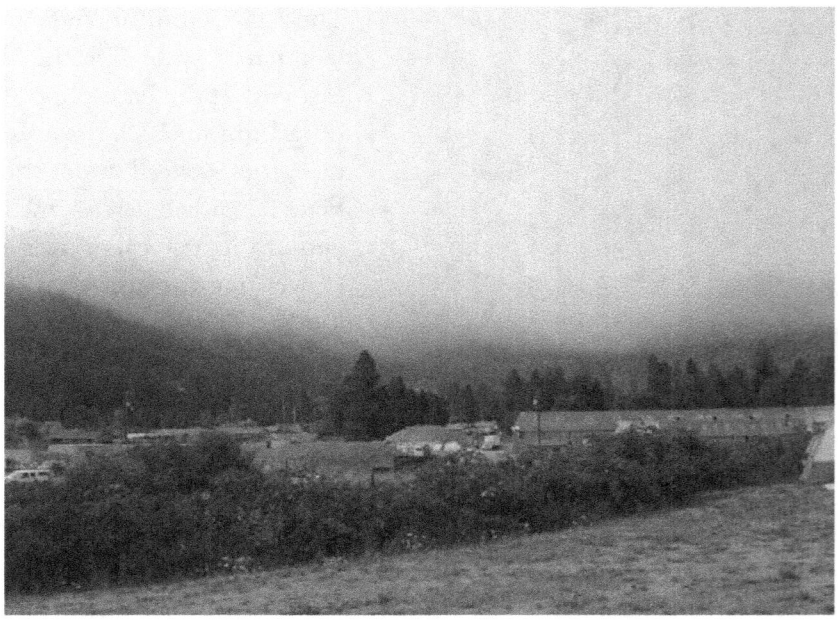

Figure 2. Early morning smoke (approximately 8:30 a.m.) in the base camp on August 13, 2008.

Figure 3. Midmorning smoke (approximately 10:00 a.m.) in the base camp on August 13, 2008.

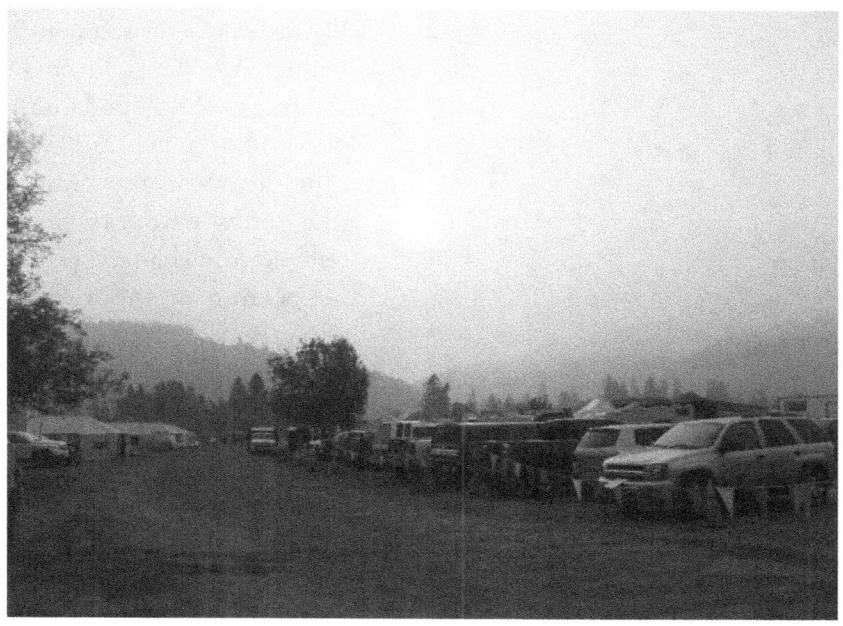

Figure 4. Early morning smoke (approximately 7:30 a.m.) in the base camp on August 14, 2008.

Carboxyhemoglobin in Blood

Over the 2-day period, 19 nonsmoking employees had COHb measurements taken. Although not directly comparable to the ACGIH BEI (end of shift, 8-hour COHb measurement of 3.5%), 3 of 19 (11%) nonsmoking employees (reefer, resources, and supply/logistics personnel) met or exceeded a COHb measurement of 3.5%, which is considered an indicator of a 25-ppm, 8-hour TWA CO exposure. One employee showed a progressive increase in COHb that exceeded 3.5% in the late evening of August 13, 2008, returned to 1% at the start of the next day, and then increased again above 3 5% during the next day's work shift. This employee had one measured peak CO concentration above the ACGIH excursion limit of 125 ppm during the late morning of August 13, 2008, but had average CO exposures below 3 ppm during the two work shifts and overnight. The other two employees with COHb readings at or above 3.5% did not have any measured CO concentrations exceeding relevant OELs. All three employees, as with all tested employees, had low average PBZ CO exposures.

Environmental Data

Figure 5 presents temperature, relative humidity, and dew point temperature data collected during the site visit. The data show that the August 13, 2008, afternoon air temperature reached 100°F, dew point temperature ranged between 50°F and 55°F, and relative humidity was consistently around 20% during the afternoon (the hottest part of the day). During the evening hours, the air temperature changed over 40°F as the August 14, 2008, morning temperature was approximately 57°F. At the end of the evaluation on August 14, 2008, the daytime air temperature was 90°F. It is important to note that the daytime relative humidity dropped to 20%, indicating an environment that many people would perceive as dry.

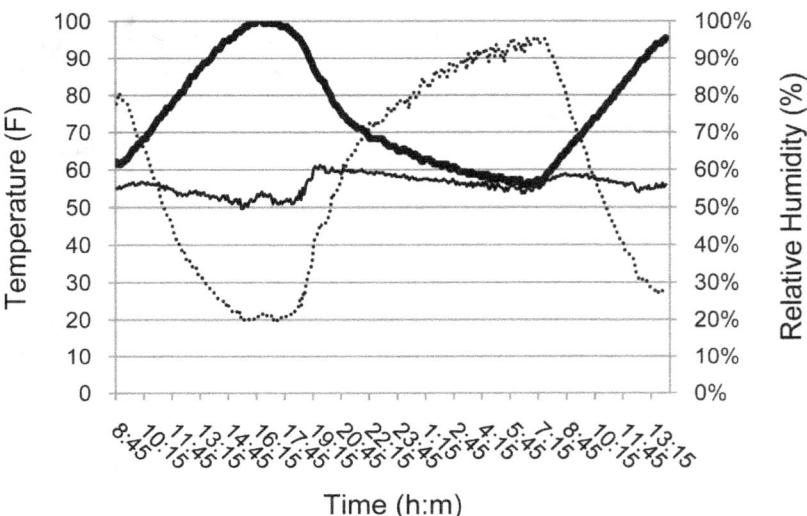

Figure 5. Outdoor environmental data collected at the base camp's north end – temperature, dew point temperature, and relative humidity measurements on August 13–14, 2008.

DISCUSSION

During our evaluation, average CO air concentrations measured on employees were low (< 3 ppm), although some base camp personnel had brief peak CO exposures exceeding relevant OELs including a few in excess of 1000 ppm. However, these elevated peak exposures were all very short duration (< 1 minute). The elevated peak CO concentrations could have been a result of the job task for the day (e.g., mechanic conducting vehicle maintenance) and/or the location of an employee in the base camp (e.g., supply area in close proximity to vehicles moving in or out of the base camp). Although there were obvious sources of CO in addition to the fires (i.e., vehicle exhaust and three 3,000-watt gas generators), most sources of power in the base camp were diesel generators, which, if maintained properly, should not emit CO at concentrations found in our peak measurements. Radio frequency signals from the use of two-way radios could have caused a spike in the signal that was recorded as a CO peak, as this is a known interference for the CO monitors [NIOSH 2000]. It was not possible to collect detailed information on the location of all base camp personnel during the day due to the size of the camp and number of base camp personnel. Thus, we were unable to correlate every activity with a particular CO concentration.

The nature of this type of work makes interpretation of our CO and COHb results difficult. Employees typically worked 16-hour shifts in the base camp, their nonwork time continues in the base camp, and CO exposure continues during the overnight hours, essentially maintaining some low level of exposure to CO for a continuous 24-hour period. This nontraditional work shift complicates comparing employee exposures to OELs established for a typical 8- to 10-hour work shift and 40-hour workweek. Additional factors – such as, a long and busy fire season, an individual's potential for numerous deployments to base camps, the varying distances from the base camp to the forest fire, many consecutive 16-hour workdays without a break (time or day off) from exposure, and the varying environmental conditions – further complicates the measurement and interpretation of potential CO exposures.

COHb measurements were for the most part consistent with ambient CO levels; that is, low COHb levels reflected low ambient CO concentrations. However, there were a few elevated COHb readings among base camp personnel. The elevated COHb readings may have been a result of an unrecognized CO source, equipment inaccuracy, unreported smoking, or operator error.

DISCUSSION
(CONTINUED)

Exposure to low ambient CO concentrations has been reported to affect multiple body systems, but most studies involved shorter periods with continuous levels of CO exposure, unlike the exposures at the base camp. There is limited evidence that volunteers exposed to CO have shown subtle brain function changes when COHb levels are about 5% [EPA 1979, 1984]. These changes in brain function involved tasks that required sustained attention or performance, such as hand-eye coordination and detection of infrequent events. Some research has found that low-level CO exposure affects exercise performance, but other studies have not found this effect. In the 1970s, COHb levels between 2.5% and 4% were found to decrease maximal exercise duration in young healthy men in the short term [Aronow and Cassidy 1975]. However, no studies have been published that have examined longer-term effects of low-level exposure to CO on exercise duration. At slightly higher levels than we found at the base camp, two researchers found that short-term CO inhalation producing a COHb of 6.9% had no significant effect on the cardiovascular or respiratory responses of young healthy men [Turner and McNicol 1993]. The levels of COHb we found among employees at the base camp have not been reported to cause the symptoms that can occur with short-term, higher levels of CO exposure. However, the combination of consecutive 16-hour work shifts, continuous exposure to forest fire smoke, and hot environmental conditions could explain headaches reported in the HHE request among some base camp personnel.

Extended work shifts themselves may result in employee stress, fatigue, decreased concentration, deteriorating performance, and other adverse effects. OSHA suggests that management should limit the amount of time employees work extended shifts and, if extended shifts are unavoidable, ensure employees have enough time for rest and recovery [OSHA 2004]. NIOSH provides additional information and guidance on their work schedule topic page "Work Schedules: Shift Work and Long Work Hours" [NIOSH 2010] and in the publication Overtime and Extended Work Shifts: Recent Findings on Illnesses, Injuries and Health Behaviors [NIOSH 2004].

DISCUSSION
(CONTINUED)

The environmental conditions measured during this evaluation indicate a potential for heat stress and strain. High temperatures may lead to heat-related illnesses if base camp personnel are working outside air-conditioned tents or trailers for extended periods. An agency-established heat awareness program is recommended for base camp personnel as a method of prevention and a continuing reminder of the potential for heat-related illness while on duty.

Although this evaluation focused on CO exposures, base camp personnel also expressed a concern about particulate exposures. Numerous studies of firefighter (less extensive for base camp personnel) exposures to wildland fire smoke and its constituents, including CO and particulates, have been published [NIOSH 1992a,b,c, 1994, 2000; Materna et al. 1992; USDA 1999, 2000a,b; Reinhardt and Ottmar 2004; Gaughan et al. 2008].

CONCLUSIONS

Although average CO concentrations measured on base camp personnel were low, peak exposures exceeding relevant OELs did occasionally occur. In most cases, COHb measurements reflected the low personal CO exposure concentrations and the low ambient CO concentrations found. Although not directly comparable to the ACGIH BEI because of 16-hour work shifts, some nonsmoking employees met or exceeded a COHb measurement of 3.5%. The combination of consecutive 16-hour work shifts, 24-hour low-level exposure to CO, exposure to other contaminants in forest fire smoke, and hot environmental conditions could result in adverse health effects among base camp personnel; efforts should be made to minimize exposures.

RECOMMENDATIONS

Based on our findings, we recommend the actions listed below to create a more healthful workplace. We encourage the agency to use a labor-management health and safety committee or working group to discuss the recommendations in this report and develop an action plan. Those involved in the work can best set priorities and assess the feasibility of our recommendations for the agency-specific situation. Our recommendations are based on the hierarchy of controls approach (refer to Appendix B: Occupational Exposure Limits and Health Effects). This approach groups actions by their likely effectiveness in reducing or removing hazards. In most cases, the preferred approach is to eliminate hazardous materials or processes and install engineering controls to reduce exposure or shield employees. Until such controls are in place, or if they are not effective or feasible, administrative measures and/or personal protective equipment may be needed.

Administrative Controls

Administrative controls are management-dictated work practices and policies to reduce or prevent exposures to workplace hazards. The effectiveness of administrative changes in work practices for controlling workplace hazards is dependent on management commitment and employee acceptance. Regular monitoring and reinforcement is necessary to ensure that control policies and procedures are not circumvented in the name of convenience or production.

1. Develop a base camp air monitoring program during a future fire season that would include particulate exposure monitoring in addition to CO.
   - Include monitoring of COHb levels in employees using a pulse CO-oximeter, exhaled breath CO analysis [ACGIH 2001], or both.
   - Refer to the previous wildland firefighter studies referenced in this report for guidance on environmental sampling methods used to evaluate exposures to CO and particulates in addition to other potential contaminants.
   - Consider developing CO and particulate action levels to reduce exposure during future fire events, taking into consideration employees' extended work shifts. For example, an action level would trigger a removal of the employee from the base camp for a designated period or relocation of the base camp to another area.

RECOMMENDATIONS
(CONTINUED)

2. Establish a heat stress awareness program and refer to the NIOSH criteria on hot work environments [NIOSH 1986]. This program should include the following components:

   - Monitoring the environmental heat in the base camp.

   - Briefing base camp personnel on the day's weather forecast and the potential for a heat alert.

   - Ensuring that, during difficult environmental conditions, personnel stay inside cooled tents or trailers as much as possible and drink fluids to remain hydrated.

   - Training employees on the hazards of heat stress, signs and symptoms of heat-related illness and first-aid procedures for treatment, and preventive measures and employee responsibilities to avoid heat stress.

   - Informing a supervisor if an employee feels weak, nauseated, excessively fatigued, confused, and/or irritable.

3. Limit the number of personnel working extended work shifts and the frequency/duration of extended work shifts. When extended work shifts are necessary, ensure adequate rest and recovery time. Refer to NIOSH and OSHA guidance on extended work shifts [NIOSH 2004; OSHA 2004].

REFERENCES

ACGIH [2001]. Documentation of threshold limit values and biological exposure indices. 7th edition. Cincinnati, OH: American Conference of Governmental Industrial Hygienists.

Aronow WS, Cassidy J [1975]. The effect of carbon monoxide on maximal treadmill exercise. A study of normal persons. Ann Intern Med 83(4):496–500.

EPA [1979]. Air quality criteria for carbon monoxide. Research Triangle Park, NC: U.S. Environmental Protection Agency, Office of Health and Environmental Assessment, Environmental Criteria and Assessment Office, EPA Report No. EPA-600/8-79-022, NTIS No. PB81-244840.

EPA [1984]. Revised evaluation of health effects associated with carbon monoxide exposure: an addendum to the 1979 EPA air quality criteria document for carbon monoxide. Research Triangle Park, NC: U.S. Environmental Protection Agency, Office of Health and Environmental Assessment, Environmental Criteria and Assessment Office, EPA Report No. EPA 600/8-83-033F, NTIS No. PB85-103471.

Gaughan DM, Cox-Ganser JM, Enright PL, Castellan RM, Wagner GR, Hobbs GR, Bledsoe TA, Siegel PD, Kreiss K, Weissman DN [2008]. Acute upper and lower respiratory effects in wildland firefighters. J Occup Environ Med 50(9):1019–1028.

Materna BL, Jones JR, Sutton PM, Rothman N, Harrison RJ [1992]. Occupational exposures in California wildland fire fighting. Am Ind Hyg Assoc J 53(1):69–76.

NIOSH [1986]. Criteria for a recommended standard: occupational exposure to hot environments, rev. Cincinnati, OH: U.S. Department of Health and Human Services, Centers for Disease Control, National Institute for Occupational Safety and Health, DHHS (NIOSH) Publication No. 86-113.

NIOSH [1992a]. Hazard evaluation and technical assistance report: U.S. Department of the Interior, National Park Service, Gallatin National Forest, Montana. By Kelly JE. Cincinnati, OH: U.S. Department of Health and Human Services, Centers for Disease Control and Prevention, National Institute for Occupational Safety and Health, NIOSH HETA Report No. 91-312-2185.

REFERENCES
(CONTINUED)

NIOSH [1992b]. Hazard evaluation and technical assistance report: U.S. Department of the Interior, National Park Service, New River Gorge National River, West Virginia. By Kelly JE. Cincinnati, OH: U.S. Department of Health and Human Services, Centers for Disease Control and Prevention, National Institute for Occupational Safety and Health, NIOSH HETA Report No. 92-045-2260.

NIOSH [1992c]. Hazard evaluation and technical assistance report: U.S. Department of the Interior, National Park Service, Yellowstone National Park, Wyoming. By Reh CM, Deitchman S. Cincinnati, OH: U.S. Department of Health and Human Services, Centers for Disease Control and Prevention, National Institute for Occupational Safety and Health, NIOSH HETA Report No. 88-320-2176.

NIOSH [1994]. Hazard evaluation and technical assistance report: U.S. Department of the Interior, National Park Service, Yosemite National Park, California. By Reh CM, Letts D, Deitchman S. Cincinnati, OH: U.S. Department of Health and Human Services, Centers for Disease Control and Prevention, National Institute for Occupational Safety and Health, NIOSH HETA Report No. 90-0365-2415.

NIOSH [2000]. Hazard evaluation and technical assistance report: Colorado Department of Public Health and Environment, Colorado. By McCammon JB, McKenzie L. Cincinnati, OH: U.S. Department of Health and Human Services, Centers for Disease Control and Prevention, National Institute for Occupational Safety and Health, NIOSH HETA Report No. 98-0173-2782.

NIOSH [2004]. Overtime and extended work shifts: recent findings on illnesses, injuries, and health behaviors. By Caruso CC, Hitchcock EM, Dick RB, Russo JM, Schmit JM. Cincinnati, OH: U.S. Department of Health and Human Services, Centers for Disease Control and Prevention, National Institute for Occupational Safety and Health, DHHS (NIOSH) Publication No. 2004-143.

NIOSH [2010]. Work schedules: shift work and long work hours. [www.cdc.gov/niosh/topics/ workschedules/]. Date accessed: April 2011.

REFERENCES
(CONTINUED)

OSHA [2004]. Extended/unusual workshifts. [www.osha.gov/ SLTC/emergencypreparedness/ guides/extended.html]. Date accessed: April 2011.

Reinhardt TE, Ottmar RD [2004]. Baseline Measurements of smoke exposure among wildland firefighters. J Occup Environ Hyg 1(9):593–606.

Turner JA, McNicol MW [1993]. The effect of nicotine and carbon monoxide on exercise performance in normal subjects. Respir Med 87(6):421–431.

USDA [1999]. Guide to monitoring smoke exposure of wildland firefighters. By Reinhardt TE, Ottmar RD, Hallett MJ. Portland, OR: U.S. Department of Agriculture, Forest Service, Pacific Northwest Research Station, Pacific Northwest General Technical Report PNW-GTR-448.

USDA [2000a]. Smoke exposure among firefighters at prescribed burns in the Pacific Northwest. By Reinhardt TE, Ottmar RD, Hanneman AJS. Portland, OR: U.S. Department of Agriculture, Forest Service, Pacific Northwest Research Station, Pacific Northwest Research Paper PNW-RP-526.

USDA [2000b]. Smoke exposure at western wildfires. By Reinhardt TE, Ottmar RD. Portland, OR: U.S. Department of Agriculture, Forest Service, Pacific Northwest Research Station, Pacific Northwest Research Paper PNW-RP-525.

USFS [2008]. Klamath National Forest. [www.fs.fed.us/r5/ klamath/about/index.shtml]. Date accessed: April 2011.

APPENDIX A: METHODS

Carbon Monoxide in Air

We measured CO air concentrations in the PBZ of base camp personnel and at GA work locations using ToxiUltra Atmospheric Monitors (Biosystems, Inc , Middletown, Connecticut) with CO sensors. All ToxiUltra CO monitors were zeroed and calibrated before each use, according to the manufacturer's recommendations. These monitors are direct-reading instruments with data-logging capabilities. The instruments were operated in the passive diffusion mode, with a 1-minute sampling interval. The instruments have a nominal range from 0 to 500 ppm with a maximum instantaneous reading of 1000 ppm.

Additional GA air samples for CO were collected using five RAE Systems AreaRAE monitors (Rae® Systems, San Jose, California). AreaRAEs are multigas monitors that measure specific substances, such as CO, using electrochemical cells. The monitors are capable of wireless operation and real-time data transfer to a base controller.

Carboxyhemoglobin in Blood

We collected noninvasive measurements of COHb on base camp personnel using a Masimo® Rad-57 signal extraction pulse CO-Oximeter™ (Masimo Corporation, Irvine, California). This instrument uses a finger sensor that emits wavelengths of light to collect and analyze physiological data and determine COHb levels. The U.S. Food and Drug Administration approves its use for the measurement of COHb. The manufacturer states the instrument measures COHb in the range of 1%–40% with an accuracy of +/- 3% [Masimo 2008]. The test is painless and takes approximately 10 to 15 seconds to perform a single reading. Unlike exhaled breath CO testing, this instrument allows noninvasive measurement of COHb without subject cooperation or effort. Pulse CO-oximetry has been shown to be a reliable method of measuring COHb [Mottram et al. 2005; Barker et al. 2006; Hampson et al. 2006; Chee et al. 2008; Suner et al. 2008; Suner and McMurdy 2009].

Environmental Data

A HOBO® Weather Station (Onset Computer Corporation, Bourne, Massachusetts) was used to collect climate information (temperature, relative humidity, dew point) at the base camp during the entire site visit. This data logger is capable of measuring and storing data for up to 15 different parameters.

References

Barker S, Curry J, Redford D, Morgan S [2006]. Measurement of carboxyhemoglobin and methemoglobin by pulse oximetry. Anesthesiology 105(5):892–897.

Chee K, Nilson D, Partridge R, Hughes A, Suner S, Sucov A, Jay G [2008]. Finding needles in a haystack: a case series of carbon monoxide poisoning detected using new technology in the emergency department. Clin Toxicol 46(5):461–469.

Hampson N, Ecker E, Scott K [2006]. Use of a noninvasive pulse CO-oximeter to measure blood carboxyhemoglobin levels in bingo players. Respir Care 51(7):758–760.

Masimo Corporation [2008]. Breakthrough noninvasive patient monitoring technologies. [www.masimo.com/]. Date accessed: April 2011.

Mottram C, Hanson L, Scanlon P [2005]. Comparison of the Masimo Rad57 pulse oximeter with SpCO technology against a laboratory CO-oximeter using arterial blood. Respir Care 50(11):1471.

Suner S, McMurdy J [2009]. Masimo Rad-57 Pulse CO-OximeterTM for noninvasive carboxyhemoglobin measurement. Expert Rev Med Devices 6(2):125–130.

Suner S, Partridge R, Sucov A, Valente J, Chee K, Hughes A, Jay G [2008]. Non-invasive pulse CO-oximetry screening in the emergency department identifies occult carbon monoxide toxicity. J Emerg Med 34(4):441–450.

APPENDIX B: OCCUPATIONAL EXPOSURE LIMITS AND HEALTH EFFECTS

In evaluating the hazards posed by workplace exposures, NIOSH investigators use both mandatory (legally enforceable) and recommended OELs for chemical, physical, and biological agents as a guide for making recommendations. OELs have been developed by federal agencies and safety and health organizations to prevent the occurrence of adverse health effects from workplace exposures. Generally, OELs suggest levels of exposure that most employees may be exposed to for up to 10 hours per day, 40 hours per week, for a working lifetime, without experiencing adverse health effects. However, not all employees will be protected from adverse health effects even if their exposures are maintained below these levels. A small percentage may experience adverse health effects because of individual susceptibility, a preexisting medical condition, and/or a hypersensitivity (allergy). In addition, some hazardous substances may act in combination with other workplace exposures, the general environment, or with medications or personal habits of the employee to produce adverse health effects even if the occupational exposures are controlled at the level set by the exposure limit. Also, some substances can be absorbed by direct contact with the skin and mucous membranes in addition to being inhaled, which contributes to the individual's overall exposure.

Most OELs are expressed as a TWA exposure. A TWA refers to the average exposure during a normal 8- to 10-hour workday. Some chemical substances and physical agents have recommended STEL or ceiling values where adverse health effects are caused by exposures over a short period. Unless otherwise noted, the STEL is a 15-minute TWA exposure that should not be exceeded at any time during a workday, and the ceiling limit is an exposure that should not be exceeded at any time.

In the United States, OELs have been established by federal agencies, professional organizations, state and local governments, and other entities. Some OELs are legally enforceable limits, while others are recommendations. The U.S. Department of Labor OSHA PELs (29 CFR 1910 [general industry]; 29 CFR 1926 [construction industry]; and 29 CFR 1917 [maritime industry]) are legal limits enforceable in workplaces covered under the Occupational Safety and Health Act of 1970. NIOSH RELs are recommendations based on a critical review of the scientific and technical information available on a given hazard and the adequacy of methods to identify and control the hazard. NIOSH RELs can be found in the NIOSH Pocket Guide to Chemical Hazards [NIOSH 2005]. NIOSH also recommends different types of risk management practices (e.g., engineering controls, safe work practices, employee education/ training, personal protective equipment, and exposure and medical monitoring) to minimize the risk of exposure and adverse health effects from these hazards. Other OELs that are commonly used and cited in the United States include the TLVs recommended by ACGIH, a professional organization, and the WEELs recommended by the American Industrial Hygiene Association, another professional organization. The TLVs and WEELs are developed by committee members of these associations from a review of the published, peer-reviewed literature. They are not consensus standards. ACGIH TLVs are considered voluntary exposure guidelines for use by industrial hygienists and others trained in this discipline "to assist in the control of health hazards" [ACGIH 2011]. WEELs have been established for some chemicals "when no other legal or authoritative limits exist" [AIHA 2010].

Outside the United States, OELs have been established by various agencies and organizations and include both legal and recommended limits. The Institut für Arbeitsschutz der Deutschen Gesetzlichen Unfallversicherung (IFA, Institute for Occupational Safety and Health of the German Social Accident Insurance) maintains a database of international OELs from European Union member states, Canada (Québec), Japan, Switzerland, and the United States. The database, available at www.dguv.de/ifa/en/gestis/limit_values/index.jsp, contains international limits for over 1,500 hazardous substances and is updated periodically.

Employers should understand that not all hazardous chemicals have specific OSHA PELs, and for some agents the legally enforceable and recommended limits may not reflect current health-based information. However, an employer is still required by OSHA to protect its employees from hazards even in the absence of a specific OSHA PEL. OSHA requires an employer to furnish employees a place of employment free from recognized hazards that cause or are likely to cause death or serious physical harm [Occupational Safety and Health Act of 1970 (Public Law 91–596, sec. 5(a)(1))]. Thus, NIOSH investigators encourage employers to make use of other OELs when making risk assessments and risk management decisions to best protect the health of their employees. NIOSH investigators also encourage the use of the traditional hierarchy of controls approach to eliminate or minimize identified workplace hazards. This includes, in order of preference, the use of (1) substitution or elimination of the hazardous agent, (2) engineering controls (e.g , local exhaust ventilation, process enclosure, dilution ventilation), (3) administrative controls (e.g., limiting time of exposure, employee training, work practice changes, medical surveillance), and (4) personal protective equipment (e.g., respiratory protection, gloves, eye protection, hearing protection). Control banding, a qualitative risk assessment and risk management tool, is a complementary approach to protecting employee health that focuses resources on exposure controls by describing how a risk needs to be managed. Information on control banding is available at http://www.cdc.gov/niosh/topics/ctrlbanding/. This approach can be applied in situations where OELs have not been established or can be used to supplement the OELs, when available.

Carbon monoxide

CO is a colorless, odorless, tasteless gas produced by incomplete burning of carbon-containing materials. The initial symptoms of CO poisoning may include headache, dizziness, drowsiness, or nausea. Symptoms may advance to vomiting, loss of consciousness, and collapse if prolonged or high exposures are encountered. If the exposure level is high, loss of consciousness may occur without other symptoms. Coma or death may occur if high exposures continue [NIOSH 1972, 1977, 1979, 2005; Proctor et al. 1988; ACGIH 2001]. The display of symptoms varies widely from individual to individual and may occur sooner in susceptible individuals, such as young or aged people, people with preexisting lung or heart disease, or those living at high altitudes.

Exposure to CO limits the ability of the blood to carry oxygen to the tissues by binding with the hemoglobin to form COHb. Once exposed, the body compensates for the reduced blood-borne oxygen by increasing cardiac output, thereby increasing blood flow to specific oxygen-demanding organs such as the brain and heart. This ability may be limited by preexisting heart or lung diseases that inhibit increased cardiac output.

Blood has an estimated 210–250 times greater affinity for CO than oxygen, thus the presence of CO in the blood can interfere with oxygen uptake and delivery to the body. Once absorbed into the bloodstream, the half-time of CO disappearance from blood (referred to as the "half-life") varies widely by individual and circumstance (e.g., removal from exposure, initial COHb concentration, partial pressure of oxygen after exposure). Under normal recovery conditions that include breathing ambient air, the half-life can be expected to range from 2 to 6.5 hours [WHO 1999]. This means that if the initial COHb level were 10%, it could be expected to drop to 5% in 2 or more hours and then to 2.5% in another 2 or more hours. If the exposed person is treated with oxygen, as happens in emergency treatment, the half-life time is decreased again by as much as 75% (or to as low as approximately 40 minutes). Delivery of oxygen under pressure (hyperbaric treatment) reduces the half-life to approximately 20 minutes.

COHb levels vary in persons without occupational exposure to CO. Nonsmokers range from less than 2% to 3%; tobacco smokers range from 5% to 20%; and commuters on urban highways can have levels of 5% or more [EPA 1991; ACGIH 2001].

Occupational Exposure Criteria

Occupational criteria for CO exposure are applicable to employees who may be at risk of CO poisoning. The occupational exposure limits noted below should not be used for interpreting general population exposures, because occupational standards are intended for healthy worker populations. The effects of CO are more pronounced in a shorter time if the person is physically active, very young, very old, or has preexisting health conditions such as lung or heart disease. Persons at extremes of age and persons with underlying health conditions may have marked symptoms and may suffer serious complications at lower levels of COHb [Kales 1993]. Standards relevant to the general population consider these factors and are listed following the evaluation criteria to aid in understanding information presented in the discussion section of this report.

Although not directly applicable to the agency 16-hour extended work shift, the NIOSH REL for CO is 35 ppm for full shift TWA exposure (up to 10 hours) [NIOSH 1992]. The NIOSH REL of 35 ppm is designed to protect workers from adverse health effects associated with COHb levels in excess of 5% [NIOSH 1972]. NIOSH has established a CO ceiling limit of 200 ppm that should never be exceeded and an IDLH value of 1200 ppm [NIOSH 1992, 2000]. An IDLH value is defined as a concentration at which an immediate or delayed threat to life exists or that would interfere with an individual's ability to escape unaided from a space.

The ACGIH recommends an 8-hour TWA TLV of 25 ppm based upon limiting shifts in COHb levels to less than 3.5%, thus minimizing adverse neurobehavioral effects, such as headache and dizziness, and to maintain cardiovascular exercise capacity [ACGIH 2001]. ACGIH also recommends that exposures never exceed five times the TLV (thus, never to exceed 125 ppm) [ACGIH 2011]. ACGIH recommends a BEI for end-of-shift blood analysis in nonsmoking workers (exposed to CO) of 3.5% COHb [ACGIH 2011]. The BEI generally indicates a concentration below which nearly all workers should not experience adverse health effects. The BEI cannot be applied to current smokers, since smokers have been shown to have COHb levels between 4% and 10% [ACGIH 2001; Tomaczewski 2002] and can exceed 15% in heavy smokers [Lauwerys and Hoet 2001].

The OSHA PEL for CO is 50 ppm for an 8-hour TWA exposure [29 CFR 1910.1000]. OSHA does not currently have a standard for extended work shifts and applies an extended work shift adjustment only to full-shift occupational lead exposures [OSHA 1997].

Health Criteria Relevant to the General Public

The EPA has promulgated a NAAQS for CO. This standard requires that ambient air contain no more than 9 ppm CO for an 8-hour TWA and 35 ppm for a 1-hour average [EPA 1991]. The NAAQS for CO was established to protect "the most sensitive members of the general population" by maintaining increases in COHb to less than 2.1%.

The WHO has recommended guideline values and periods of TWA exposures related to CO exposure in the general population [WHO 1999]. WHO guidelines are intended to ensure that COHb levels not exceed 2.5% when a normal subject engages in light or moderate exercise. Those guidelines are 100 mg/m3 (87 ppm) for 15 minutes, 60 mg/m3 (52 ppm) for 30 minutes, 30 mg/m3 (26 ppm) for 1 hour, and 10 mg/m3 (9 ppm) for 8 hours.

References

ACGIH [2001]. Documentation of threshold limit values and biological exposure indices. 7th edition. Cincinnati, OH: American Conference of Governmental Industrial Hygienists.

ACGIH [2011]. 2011 TLVs® and BEIs®: threshold limit values for chemical substances and physical agents and biological exposure indices. Cincinnati, OH: American Conference of Governmental Industrial Hygienists.

AIHA [2010]. AIHA 2010 Emergency response planning guidelines (ERPG) & workplace environmental exposure levels (WEEL) handbook. Fairfax, VA: American Industrial Hygiene Association.

CFR. Code of Federal Regulations. Washington, DC: U.S. Government Printing Office, Office of the Federal Register.

EPA [1991]. Air quality criteria for carbon monoxide. Publication No. EPA-600/8-90/045F. Washington, DC: U.S. Environmental Protection Agency.

Kales SN [1993] Carbon monoxide intoxication. American Family Physician 48(6):1100–1104.

Lauwerys RR, Hoet P [2001]. Industrial chemical exposure: guidelines for biological monitoring. 3rd ed. Lewis Publishers (CRC Press LLC), Boca Raton, Florida. pp. 474–477.

NIOSH [1972]. Criteria for a recommended standard: occupational exposure to carbon monoxide. Cincinnati, OH: U.S. Department of Health, Education, and Welfare, Health Services and Mental Health Administration, National Institute for Occupational Safety and Health, DHEW (NIOSH) Publication No. 73-11000.

NIOSH [1977]. Occupational diseases: a guide to their recognition. Rev. ed. Cincinnati, OH: U.S. Department of Health, Education, and Welfare, Center for Disease Control, National Institute for Occupational Safety and Health, DHEW (NIOSH) Publication No. 77-181.

NIOSH [1979]. A guide to work-relatedness of disease. Rev. ed. Cincinnati, OH: U.S. Department of Health, Education, and Welfare, Center for Disease Control, National Institute for Occupational Safety and Health, DHEW (NIOSH) Publication No. 79-116.

NIOSH [1992]. Recommendations for occupational safety and health: compendium of policy documents and statements. Cincinnati, OH: U.S. Department of Health and Human Services, Centers for Disease Control and Prevention, National Institute for Occupational Safety and Health, DHHS (NIOSH) Publication No. 92-100.

NIOSH [2000]. Documentation for immediately dangerous to life or health concentrations. In: NIOSH Pocket guide to chemical hazards and other databases. Cincinnati, OH: U.S. Department of Health and Human Services, Centers for Disease Control and Prevention, National Institute for Occupational Safety and Health, DHHS (NIOSH) Publication No. 2000-130.

NIOSH [2005]. NIOSH pocket guide to chemical hazards. Cincinnati, OH: U.S. Department of Health and Human Services, Centers for Disease Control and Prevention, National Institute for Occupational Safety and Health, DHHS (NIOSH) Publication No. 2005-149. [http://www.cdc.gov/niosh/npg/]. Date accessed: April 2011.

OSHA [1997]. Standard interpretation: calculation methods used under the air contaminants standard for extended workshifts. [www.osha.gov/pls/oshaweb/owadisp.show_document?p_table=INTERPRETATIONS&p_id=22333]. Date accessed: April 2011.

Proctor NH, Hughes JP, Fischman ML [1988]. Chemical hazards of the workplace. Philadelphia, PA: J.B. Lippincott Company.

Tomaczewski C [2002]. Ch. 97 Carbon Monoxide. In: Goldfrank L, Flomenbaum N, Lewin N, et al., eds. Goldfrank's toxicologic emergencies. 7th ed. New York: McGraw-Hill, pp. 1478–1491.

WHO [1999]. Environmental health criteria 213-carbon monoxide. Second ed. Geneva, Switzerland: World Health Organization, ISBN 92 4 157213 2 (NLM classification: QV 662), ISSN 0250-863X.

APPENDIX C: TABLES

Table C1. Base camp – personal breathing zone CO concentration averages (ppm) and peaks (ppm) from August 13–14, 2008.

ID	Job	1st Shift		Overnight		Partial 2nd shift	
		Sample Time (military)	CO Avg. (Peak)	Sample Time (military)	CO Avg. (Peak)	Sample Time (military)	CO Avg. (Peak)
73	Caterer	1201–2100	3.3 (107)	2141–0800	0.12 (37)	0800–1157	0.78 (3.3)
17	Caterer	0627–2105	3.1 (57)	2135–0600	5.7 (> 1000)	0600–1157	2.4 (28)
16	Caterer	0941–2200	1.4 (22)	2200–0600	1.6 (4.6)	0600–1153	3.2 (26)
33	CMD	0749–2300	0.85 (7.1)	2300–0600	1.2 (2.2)	0600–1322	2.6 (74)
31	CMD	0739–2230	1.3 (12)	2230–0630	0.94 (2.9)	0630–1324	1.3 (4.0)
34	COMM	0810–2205	4.2 (> 1000)	0001–0819	1.1 (15)	—	
53	COMM	0753–2230	1.4 (15)	2230–0600	1.8 (4.2)	0600–1107	2.4 (8.6)
29	Mechanic	0703–2200	5.6 (423)	2200–0600	2.2 (7.3)	0600–1224	3.3 (72)
19	Mechanic	0652–2039	3.9 (> 1000)	—		0631–1224	3.0 (29)
35	Medical	0815–2200	2.7 (49)	2200–0600	1.3 (3.9)	0600–1315	1.5 (8.0)
51	Reefer	0535–2100	4.0 (> 1000)	2100–0605	0.24 (22)	—	
15	Reefer	0535–2013	1.9 (19)	—		—	
74	Reefer	0535–2100	1.8 (15)	2100–0746	0.35 (8.6)	—	
32	Resource	0749–2200	2.3 (141)	2200–0600	0.57 (5.8)	0600–1208	1.9 (15)
30	Supply/ Logistics	0735–2200	1.1 (8.6)	2200–0600	1.4 (5.5)	0600–1238	2.0 (15)
18	Supply	1029–2200	1.5 (45)	2200–0600	2.3 (80)	0600–1345	3.0 (38)
36	Supply	2043–2200	1.2 (5.0)	2200–0600	1.3 (11)	0600–1337	3.2 (128)
37	Supply	0835–2200	0.50 (11)	2200–0600	2.3 (3.5)	0600–1318	2.8 (55)
41	Weed Wash	—		—		0839–1227	5.4 (40)

Table C2. Base camp – general area CO concentration averages (ppm) and peaks (ppm) from August 13–14, 2008.

Location	Sample Time (military)*	CO Avg. (Peak) Begin–2200	CO Avg. (Peak) 2200–0500	CO Avg. (Peak) 0500–End	CO Avg. (Peak) Overall
RAE Systems AreaRAE monitors					
North Camp Area	0546–1231	0.52 (2.9)	0.01 (0.80)	0.78 (3.3)	0.48 (3.3)
Security Area (South)	0558–1231	0.24 (3.8)	0.01 (0.20)	0.21 (2.2)	0.18 (3.8)
East Camp Area	0546–0807†	0.49 (16)	0.07 (20)	0.0 (0.0)	0.34 (20)
Operations Center Area (West)	0558–1231	1.2 (3.6)	0.51 (1.8)	1.5 (3.5)	1.1 (3.6)
Shower and Kitchen (Middle of Camp)	0558–1231	0.02 (1.0)	0.0 (0.20)	0.03 (0.30)	0.02 (1.0)
ToxiUltra Atmospheric Monitors					
Agency Representatives Tent	0754–1430	2.0 (5.0)	0.0 (1.0)	2.0 (5.0)	1.0 (5.0)
Mobile Mapping Service Trailer	0745–1209	1.8 (13)	0.71 (2.9)	1.0 (2.3)	1.3 (13)
Logistics Trailer	0747–1210	2.2 (7.8)	2.9 (5.2)	3.4 (10)	2.7 (10)
Food Trailer	0750–1213	1.3 (8.6)	3.8 (52)	2.7 (9.5)	2.3 (52)
Sleeping Trailer	1912–0830‡	2.5 (4.0)	2.2 (3.0)	2.4 (3.7)	2.3 (4.0)
Laundry Trailer	0805–1215	1.2 (3.7)	2.7 (4.0)	3.6 (6.1)	2.2 (6.1)
Communication Unit Tent	0803–1208	0.51 (2.1)	0.95 (1.9)	1.6 (3.1)	1.6 (3.1)
Facilities Tent	0816–1207	1.2 (14)	1.2 (1.8)	1.8 (8.8)	1.4 (14)

* = Time begins on August 13, 2008, and ends on August 14, 2008.

† = Memory card full. No additional data collected after 0807 on August 14, 2008.

‡ = Only collected data during the overnight period while occupied by base camp personnel.

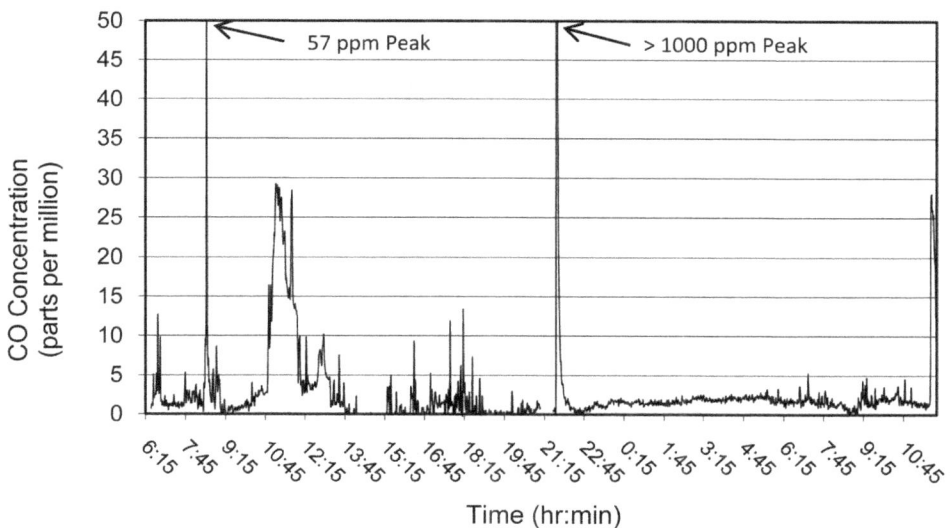

Figure D1. Caterer (ID 17) real-time CO concentrations on August 13–14, 2008, at the base camp.

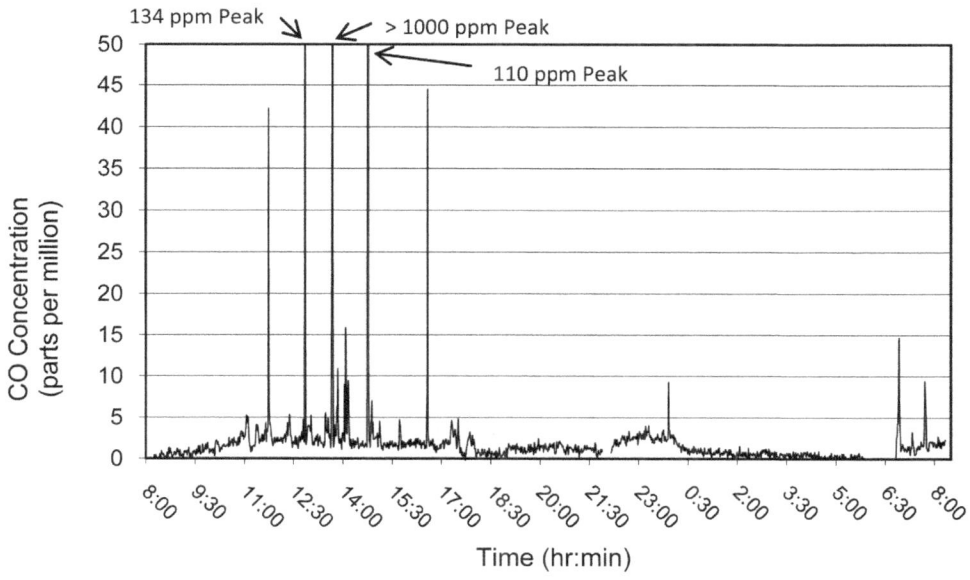

Figure D2. COMM (ID 34) real-time CO concentrations on August 13–14, 2008, at the base camp.

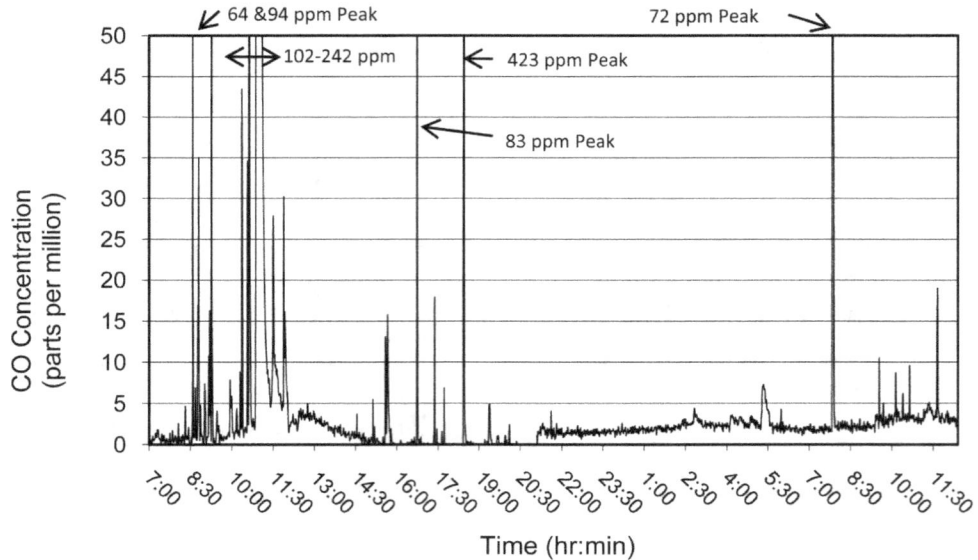

Figure D3. Mechanic (ID 29) real-time CO concentrations on August 13–14, 2008, at the base camp.

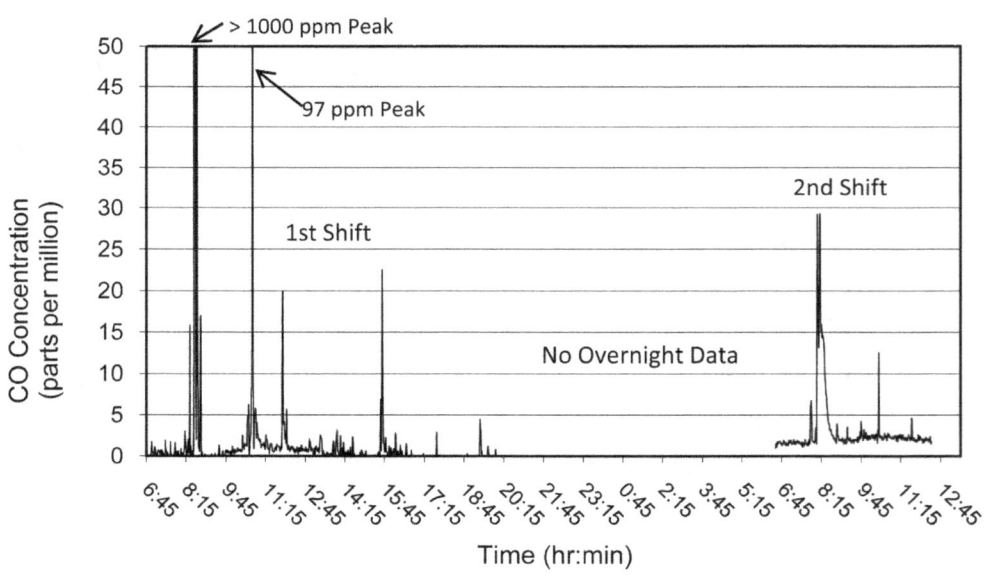

Figure D4. Mechanic (ID 19) real-time CO concentrations on August 13–14, 2008, at the base camp.

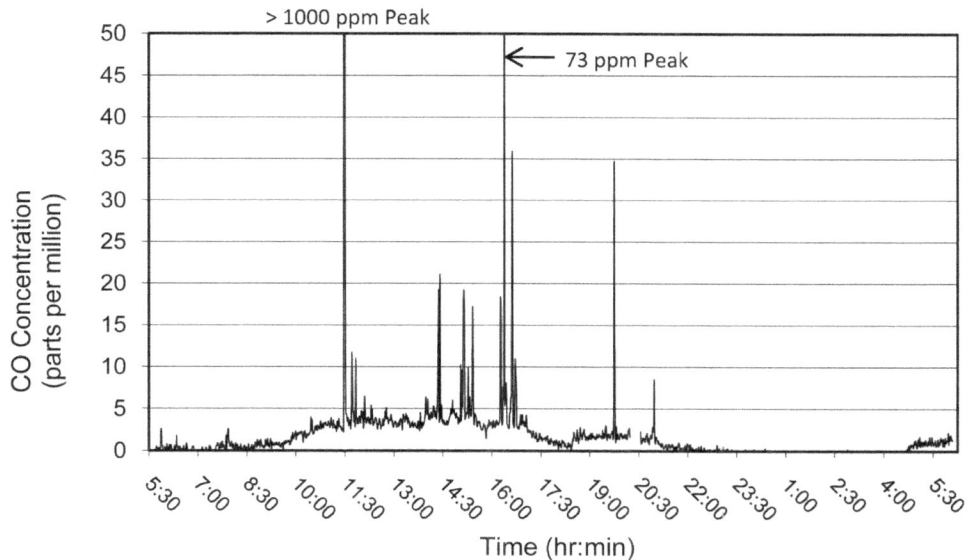

Figure D5. Reefer (ID 51) real-time CO concentrations on August 13–14, 2008, at the base camp.

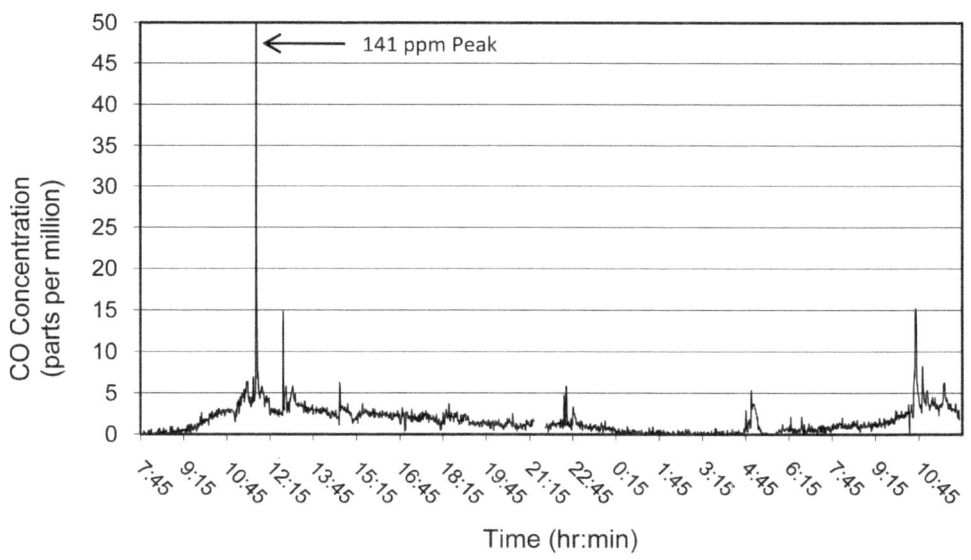

Figure D6. Resources (ID 32) real-time CO concentrations on August 13–14, 2008, at the base camp.

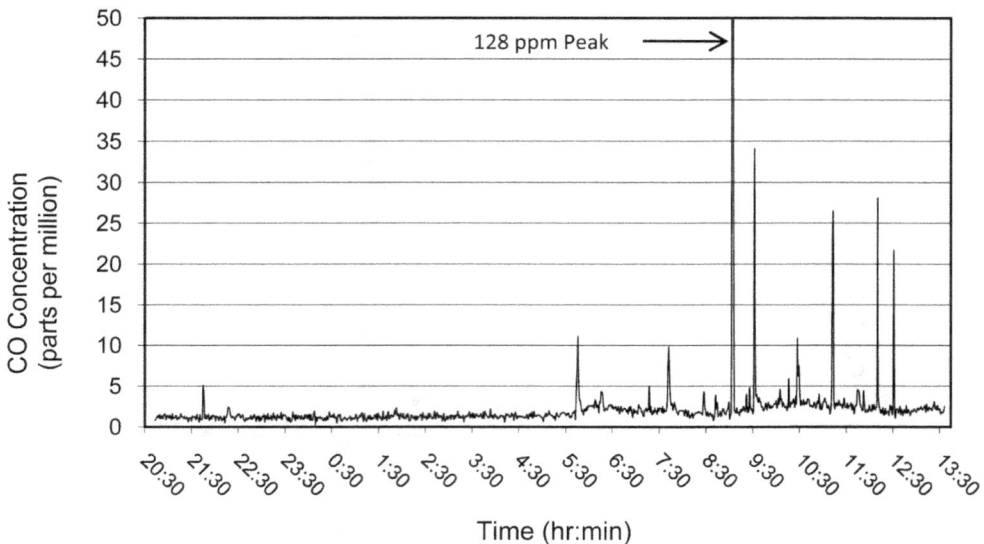

Figure D7. Supply (ID 36) real-time CO concentrations on August 13–14, 2008, at the base camp.

ACKNOWLEDGMENTS AND AVAILABILITY OF REPORT

The Hazard Evaluations and Technical Assistance Branch (HETAB) of the National Institute for Occupational Safety and Health (NIOSH) conducts field investigations of possible health hazards in the workplace. These investigations are conducted under the authority of Section 20(a)(6) of the Occupational Safety and Health Act of 1970, 29 U.S.C. 669(a)(6), which authorizes the Secretary of Health and Human Services, following a written request from any employer or authorized representative of employees, to determine whether any substance normally found in the place of employment has potentially toxic effects in such concentrations as used or found. HETAB also provides, upon request, technical and consultative assistance to federal, state, and local agencies; labor; industry; and other groups or individuals to control occupational health hazards and to prevent related trauma and disease.

The findings and conclusions in this report are those of the authors and do not necessarily represent the views of NIOSH. Mention of any company or product does not constitute endorsement by NIOSH. In addition, citations to websites external to NIOSH do not constitute NIOSH endorsement of the sponsoring organizations or their programs or products. Furthermore, NIOSH is not responsible for the content of these websites. All Web addresses referenced in this document were accessible as of the publication date.

This report was prepared by Robert E. McCleery, Anthony Almazan, and Chad H. Dowell of HETAB, Division of Surveillance, Hazard Evaluations and Field Studies, and John Snawder of the Biomonitoring and Health Assessment Branch, Division of Applied Research and Technology. Medical field assistance and support was provided by Elena Page and Bruce Bernard. Technical support was provided by Dino Mattorano of the U.S. Environmental Protection Agency. Health communication assistance was provided by Stefanie Evans. Editorial assistance was provided by Cathy Rotunda. Desktop publishing was performed by Greg Hartle.

This page left intentionally blank.

This page left intentionally blank.

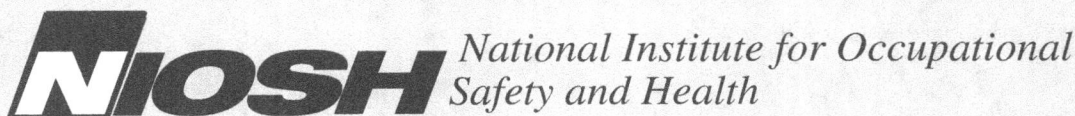

National Institute for Occupational Safety and Health

Delivering on the Nation's promise: Safety and health at work for all people through research and prevention.

To receive NIOSH documents or information about occupational safety and health topics, contact NIOSH at:

1-800-CDC-INFO (1-800-232-4636)

TTY: 1-888-232-6348

E-mail: cdcinfo@cdc.gov

or visit the NIOSH web site at: **www.cdc.gov/niosh.**

For a monthly update on news at NIOSH, subscribe to NIOSH eNews by visiting **www.cdc.gov/niosh/eNews.**

SAFER • HEALTHIER • PEOPLE™